THE 50 RECIPES ON ITALIAN VEGETARIAN SWEETS AND DESSERTS

The Latest Cookbook On The 50 Most Popular Dessert Recipes Of The Vegetarian People, From Cookies To Cakes Up To Ice Cream. If You Love Sweets And You Are Vegetarian These Recipes Are For You Easy To Prepare And Tasty To Eat.

Alberto Garofano

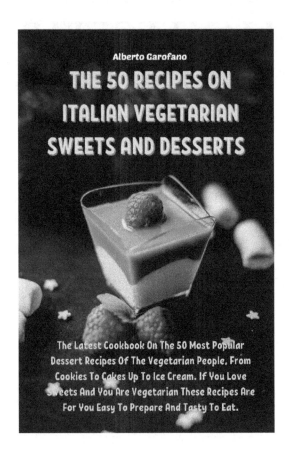

Alberto Garofano

THE 50 RECIPES ON ITALIAN VEGETARIAN SWEETS AND DESSERTS

The Latest Cookbook On The 50 Most Popular
Dessert Recipes Of The Vegetarian People, From
Cookies To Cakes Up To Ice Cream. If You Love
Sweets And You Are Vegetarian These Recipes Are
For You Easy To Prepare And Tasty To Eat.

Table Of Contents

The information in the following pages is broadly considered a truthful and accurate account of facts and as such, any inattention, use, or misuse of the information in question by the reader will render any resulting actions solely under their purview. There are no scenarios in which the publisher or the original author of this work can be in any fashion deemed liable for any hardship or damages that may befall them after undertaking information described herein.

Additionally, the information in the following pages is intended only for informational purposes and should thus be thought of as universal. As befitting its nature, it is presented without assurance regarding its prolonged validity or interim quality. Trademarks that are mentioned are done without written consent and can in no way be considered an endorsement from the trademark holder.

★ 55% OFF for BookStore NOW at $ 30,95 instead of $ 41,95! ★

The Latest Cookbook On The 50 Most Popular

Dessert Recipes Of The Vegetarian People,

From Cookies To Cakes Up To Ice Cream. If

You Love Sweets And You Are Vegetarian

These Recipes Are For You Easy To Prepare

And Tasty To Eat.

Buy is NOW and let your Customers get addicted to this amazing book!

INTRODUCTION

The vegetarian diet in Italy is spreading widely both for the ease with which vegetables are found in the markets and because they have always been present in the Mediterranean diet. Furthermore, in recent years, with the progressive increase of the world population and the continuous exploitation of the earth's resources, feeding models are being enhanced that have a low environmental impact and can be used for a long time. From these assumptions, diets are born that partially or completely avoid foods of animal origin: the vegetarian diet that does not involve the consumption of meat and fish, molluscs and crustaceans, but allows, in different ways, the consumption of eggs. And dairy products; the vegan diet which, on the other hand, eliminates all products of animal origin.

Following the indications contained in the Guidelines for healthy eating, the vegetarian diet can be formulated to meet the needs of a healthy adult:

- Eat more portions of vegetables and fresh fruit every day
- Increase the consumption of legumes , both fresh and dried
- regularly consume bread, pasta, rice and other cereals , preferably wholemeal
- Eat moderate amounts of fats and oils used for seasoning and cooking. Above all, limit fats of

animal origin (butter, lard, lard, cream, etc.) to season foods and prefer fats of vegetable origin: extra virgin olive oil and seed oils, preferably raw

- Consume eggs and milk that contain good organic quality proteins. If you drink a lot of milk, preferably choose the skim or semi-skim one which, however, maintains its calcium and vitamin content
- Eat cheeses in moderate quantities because in addition to proteins they contain high amounts of fat. For this reason it is advisable to choose the leaner ones, or eat smaller portions
- Limit foods rich in fat, salt and sugar such as creams, chocolate, chips, biscuits, sweets, ice cream, cakes and puddings to special occasions

The Elements That Cannot Be Missing In A Vegetarian Diet

The first thing to watch out for is to follow a diet that is as varied as possible. Some nutrients are present in small amounts in vegetables or are less easily absorbed by the body than those from meat or fish. However, most vegetarians generally do not have ailments due to nutrient deficiencies if they take care to include certain foods in their diet:

- Legumes combined with cereals, to ensure the availability, in addition to significant quantities of starch and fiber, of essential nutrients characteristic of meat, fish and eggs, such as iron, proteins of good biological quality, micronutrients

- Foods obtained from wholemeal flours (and not with the simple addition of bran or other fibers) which, in addition to starch and fiber, contain good amounts of calcium, iron and B vitamins

If not formulated correctly, the vegetarian diet can be deficient in essential nutrients. Those who follow it need to make sure they get sufficient amounts of iron and vitamin B12 with their food.

Plant Sources Of Iron

Vegetarians may have less iron in their body stores than people who also eat meat. It is therefore important to know the foods, suitable for vegetarians, which contain a good amount of iron:

- Eggs
- Legumes (especially lentils)
- Dried fruit
- Pumpkin seeds
- Vegetables (especially dark green ones)
- Whole grain bread
- Plant Sources of Vitamin B12

Vitamin B12 is needed for growth, cell repair, and overall health. It is found, in nature, only in products of animal origin such as, for example, meat, fish, shellfish, eggs and dairy products. If you eat these foods regularly, you are likely to be getting enough of them. However, if you only eat small amounts of foods of animal origin, or if you avoid them altogether, it is important to include certain sources of vitamin B12 in your diet:

- Milk
- Cheese
- Eggs

If the amount of vitamin B12 introduced in the diet is insufficient to meet the body's needs, it is advisable to also use foods in which it is added (fortified foods) such as:

- Fortified breakfast cereals
- Fortified soy products
- Plant sources of omega-3

The omega-3 fatty acids are found mainly in oily fish, fresh tuna and salmon. Plant sources of omega-3 fatty acids include:

- Flax seed
- Rapeseed oil
- Soybean oil and soy-based foods (such as tofu)
- Nuts

Being Vegetarian In Particular Conditions

Those who wish to follow a vegetarian diet during childhood, pregnancy, advanced age or in conjunction with illnesses, must rely on a doctor or nutritionist, because in such conditions their needs for nutrients may vary. For example, during pregnancy and breastfeeding, women following a vegetarian diet need to ensure that the amounts of vitamins and minerals in their diet are sufficient to ensure that their baby can grow healthily. While growing up, the parent must ensure that the child eats a very varied diet to meet the nutritional needs he needs.

START

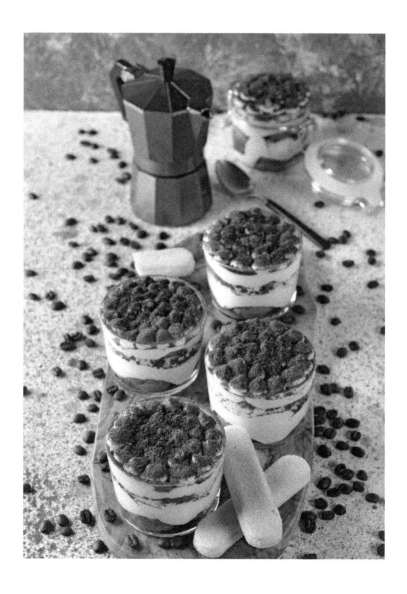

CLASSIC TIRAMISU

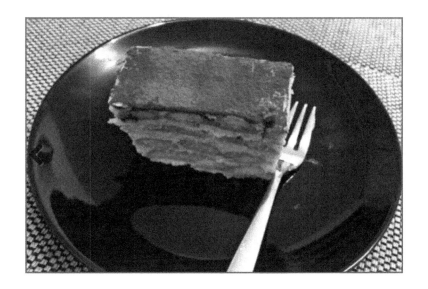

Servings:6

INGREDIENTS

- 60 Pc Ladyfingers
- 500 G Mascarpone
- 4 Pc Eggs
- 100 G Icing sugar
- 125 ml coffee
- 2 cl rum

- 6 Tbsp Cocoa for sprinkling

PREPARATION

1. For the tiramisu, the yolk and egg white are separated and placed in different bowls.
2. The egg whites are beaten with a hand mixer or food processor until stiff.
3. Then mix the yolks in the other bowl with the icing sugar to a frothy mass.
4. Next stir the mascarpone into the yolk mixture and then fold in the snow.
5. Mix the coffee and rum in a shallow bowl or plate and soak the ladyfingers in it one after the other.
6. Then alternately layer the ladyfingers and mascarpone mixture in a mold - finish with the mascarpone cream.
7. Now put the tiramisu in the refrigerator for at least 2.5 - 3 hours.
8. Sprinkle with cocoa before serving and garnish with fresh berries if desired.

BASIC PANNA COTTA RECIPE

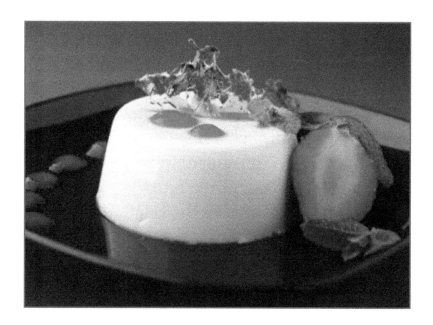

Serevings:4

INGREDIENTS

- 0.5 l Whipped cream
- 1 Pc Vanilla pod
- 5 Bl gelatin
- 40 G sugar

PREPARATION

1. Soak the gelatin in cold water. Slit the vanilla pod lengthways and scrape out the vanilla pulp.
2. In a saucepan, briefly bring the whipped cream with the vanilla pulp, the scraped out vanilla pods and the sugar to the boil and simmer gently for about 3-5 minutes.
3. Remove the saucepan from the stove and pour the hot liquid through a sieve.
4. Now take the gelatine out of the cold water, squeeze it out well and add it to the still hot, sieved mixture - stir until the gelatine has completely dissolved.
5. Fill the panna cotta mixture into small molds to turn out and place in the refrigerator for at least 4 hours.

TIRAMISU

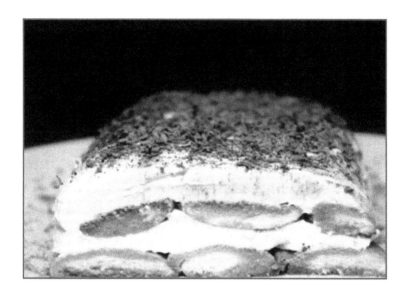

Serevings:4

INGREDIENTS
- 3 Pc Eggs
- 60 G Icing sugar
- 250 G Mascarpone
- 3 Tbsp Rum or coganc or coffee liqueur
- 150 ml espresso
- 180 G Ladyfingers
- 10 G unsweetened cocoa powder
- 1 Pc Lemon, grated zest
-

PREPARATION

1. For the Italian tiramisu, first separate the eggs and beat the egg yolks with half of the sugar in a bowl until frothy.
2. Now add the mascarpone, grated lemon zest and 3 tablespoons of rum or cognac or coffee liqueur and stir everything into a thick cream. The alcohol can of course also be left out.
3. Then beat the egg white until stiff and fold into the mascarpone cream.
4. Mix the hot espresso with the rest of the sugar and allow to cool.
5. Turn half of the sponge fingers in the cooled espresso and place in a baking dish.
6. The lady fingers should be moist but still firm. Then spread half of the mascarpone cream over it and smooth it out.
7. Now soak the remaining sponge fingers in the rest of the espresso and place on the cream.
8. Finally, spread the rest of the mascarpone over it and smooth it out.
9. Place the tiramisu in the refrigerator for at least 6 hours or overnight and sprinkle with cocoa powder before serving.

TIRAMISU WITH QIMIQ

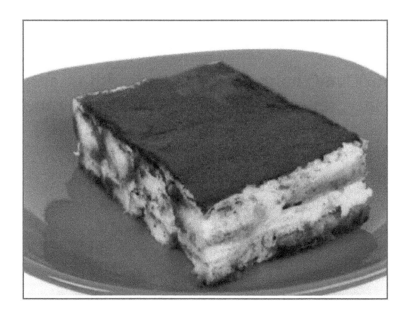

Serevings:4

INGREDIENTS

- 300 G QimiQ
- 125 G Mascarpone
- 0.125 l milk
- 1 Tbsp Dissolving coffee powder
- 90 G Fine crystal sugar
- 1 Pk vanilla sugar
- 1 cups Obers
- 45 Pc Ladyfingers

- 0.125 l coffee
- 5 Tbsp rum
- 1 prize Cocoa powder for sprinkling

PREPARATION

1. Stir QimiQ until smooth and mix with sugar, coffee, coffee powder, milk, mascarpone, rum and vanilla sugar.
2. Beat the top and fold in.
3. Line a mold with cling film, start with the cream, and then lay out alternately with the ladyfingers.
4. Finish with ladyfingers.
5. Let it steep in the refrigerator (at least 6 hours). Overturn on a plate, remove the foil and cover with cocoa.

ITALIAN PANNA COTTA

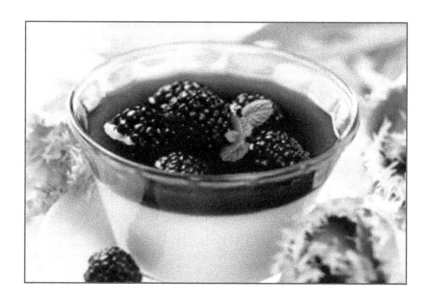

Serevings:4

INGREDIENTS

- 5 Bl   gelatin
- 50 G sugar
- 2 Pc Vanilla
- 200 ml Whipped cream
- 300 ml milk

PREPARATION

1. For this panna cotta recipe, first soak the gelatine in a little cold water. Cut the vanilla pods open on one side and scrape out the vanilla pulp.

2. In a saucepan, slowly bring the milk with the whipped cream, the scraped out vanilla pods, the vanilla pulp and the sugar to the boil and simmer over low heat for about 15 minutes.

3. Then fish out the vanilla pods and then slowly stir the squeezed out gelatine leaves into the pot, stirring constantly until they have dissolved.

4. Then pour the still warm mass into glasses bowls and let it cool down. Leave in the refrigerator for about 2 hours, garnish with a strawberry sauce and any fruit in the glass and serve.

5. The panna cotta can of course also be turned out of the glasses bowls onto a plate (hold the glass briefly in hot water).

SIMPLE COFFEE-FLAVORED TIRAMISU

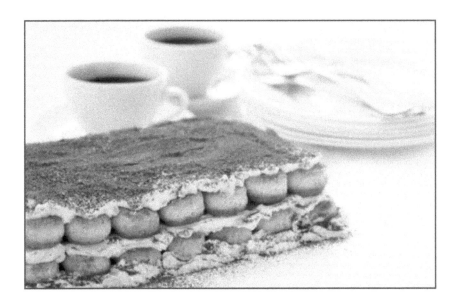

Serevings:4

INGREDIENTS

- 200 G Ladyfingers
- 250 G Mascarpone
- 2 Pc Eggs, separated (egg yolks & albumen)
- 75 G sugar
- 5 Tbsp Amaretto
- 120 ml Coffee, strongly boiled
- 3 Bl   gelatin
- 1 prize Cocoa powder

- 1 prize salt
- 0.5 Pc Lemon (zest of it)
-

PREPARATION

1. In a bowl, beat the egg yolks with the sugar until frothy.
2. Then stir in the mascarpone and the grated lemon zest.
3. In another bowl, beat the egg white with a pinch of salt and fold into the mascarpone cream.
4. Put the coffee in a shallow bowl, sweeten a little with sugar and soak the ladyfingers in it. Line the bottom of a form with the soaked ladyfingers.
5. The cream is now spread over the lady fingers. Then put another layer with soaked-up lady fingers and put the rest of the cream on top again - layers until there is no more cream. Finish with ladyfingers at the end. Sprinkle with cocoa.
6. To cool down, the mold has to be in the refrigerator for about 3 hours.

LOW CARB TIRAMISU

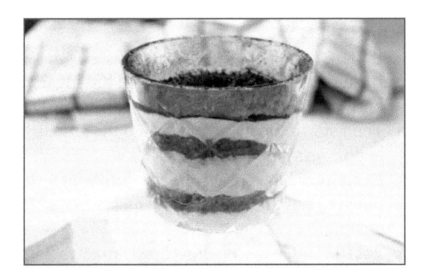

Servings:4

INGREDIENTS

- 1 Cup Coffee (fresh espresso)
- 2 Tbsp Cocoa for sprinkling

for the cream
- 500 G Mascarpone
- 3 Tbsp Sugar (e.g. xylitol or erythritol)
- 3 Pcegg yolk

for the dough

- 100 G Ground almonds
- 5 Pc Eggs
- 2 Tbsp Sugar (e.g. xylitol or erythritol)
-

PREPARATION

1. For what is probably the most famous Italian dessert, first prepare the dough. Separate the eggs and beat the egg whites in a bowl until stiff.
2. In another bowl, mix the egg yolks with the sugar and the almonds well and then carefully fold them into the egg whites.
3. Place the dough on a baking sheet and bake at 180 degrees (top / bottom heat) in a preheated oven for 20 minutes.
4. Let the dough cool down and cut out the appropriate pieces for the desired shape (glasses, casserole dish, ...). Dip the pieces in coffee (preferably espresso) and use them to lay out the bottom of the mold.
5. For the cream, mix the egg yolks with the sugar and mascarpone in a bowl. Depending on your taste, you can add a little amaretto aroma or coffee.
6. For the first layer, spread half of the mascarpone cream approx. 2 cm thick on the pieces of dough, place pieces of dough soaked

with coffee on top of the cream and finally spread the cream on top again.

7. Let the tiramisu stand in the refrigerator overnight and sprinkle with cocoa powder before serving.

PANNA COTTA WITH RASPBERRY SAUCE

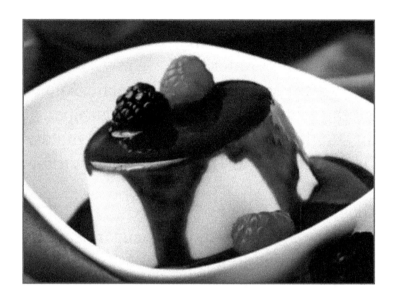

Servings:4

INGREDIENTS

- 500 G Quimiq
- 2 Tbsp sugar
- 1 Pc Vanilla pod
- 4 Bl gelatin
- 100 ml milk

For the sauce
- 500 G Raspberries
- 80 G Icing sugar
- 1 shot Lemon juice

PREPARATION

1. Bring the quimiq, milk, sugar and vanilla pod to the boil, reduce the heat, and reduce the liquid to approx. 50 milliliters.
2. Soak gelatin in water.
3. Remove the saucepan from the plate, squeeze out the gelatine and stir into the saucepan. (Stir constantly) Pour into the cold rinsed molds. Cover and leave to set in the refrigerator for 3-4 hours.
4. The raspberry sauce:
5. Mix the raspberries and icing sugar, leave to stand for about 30 minutes.
6. Puree everything, strain through a sieve, add lemon juice and use it to decorate the panna cotta.

CROSTATA

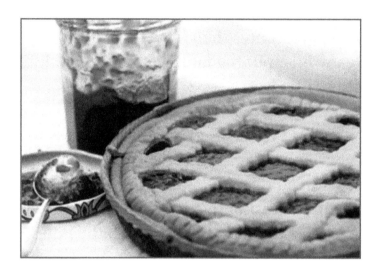

Servings:6

INGREDIENTS

- 200 G butter
- 1 Glass Jam of your choice
- 400 G Flour
- 200 G sugar
- 2 Pc Eggs
- 1 prize salt

PREPARATION

1. Mix the flour, sugar, butter and salt together, add the eggs and continue kneading the dough for a few minutes then let it rest.
2. Meanwhile, put the jam in a bowl and dilute it with a little water.
3. Divide the dough.
4. Roll up 3/4 of the dough in a round cake tin (22cm) (about 1/2 cm high), make a border, then spread the jam on the rolled out dough.
5. Roll up the rest of the dough and cut into strips, then place them on the cake with the jam so that a grid pattern is created.
6. Now bake the cake in the oven at around 180 degrees for 40 minutes, when the dough is browned, the cake is ready.

CANTUCCINI

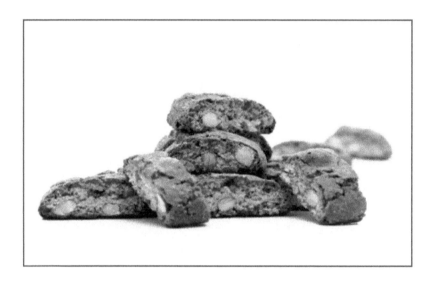

Servings:24

INGREDIENTS

- 1 TL baking powder
- 280 G Almonds
- 500 G Flour
- 1 prize salt
- 300 G sugar
- 3 Pc yolk
- 2 Pc Eggs
- 1 Pc Egg for brushing
- 2 Pk vanilla sugar

- 30 G butter

PREPARATION

1. For the cantuccini, first preheat the oven to 190 ° C. Roast the (peeled / skinless) almonds briefly in a pan without fat / oil and let them cool.
2. Now it's time to make the dough - whip the sugar with the eggs with a hand mixer until thick and creamy (at least 5 minutes).
3. Mix the flour, baking powder and salt with a spoon and then gradually stir into the egg mixture.
4. Now add the roasted, cooled almonds - knead everything well and cover the dough in the refrigerator for 30 minutes.
5. Then divide the dough into 3 equal pieces and form 3 rolls of equal length from them. The rolls are placed on a baking sheet lined with baking paper.
(Provide enough space in each case, something will open up).
6. Then brush the sticks with beaten egg and bake in the oven for approx. 15 minutes on top and bottom heat until light brown.
7. Let the dough rolls cool down and cut diagonally into 2-3 cm thick slices. Now these pieces are distributed again on the baking sheet

and baked again at 170 ° C for about 10
minutes.
8. Let the finished cantuccini cool down and put
them in the cookie jar.

ZABAGLIONE

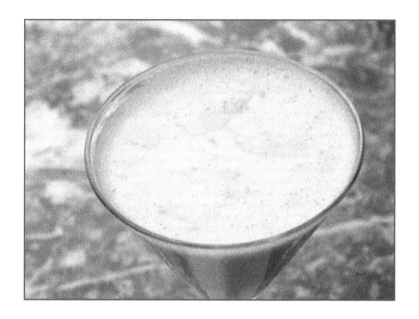

Servings:3

INGREDIENTS

- 50 G sugar
- 1 TL vanilla sugar
- 0.125 l Marsala wine
- 1 Pc Egg yolk
- 1 prize salt

PREPARATION

In a bowl, stir the egg yolks with sugar, salt and
vanilla sugar until frothy.
Gradually stir in the marsala.
Beat in a hot water bath until a brownish foam forms.
Fill into glass bowls immediately and serve.

ITALIAN ICE CREAM

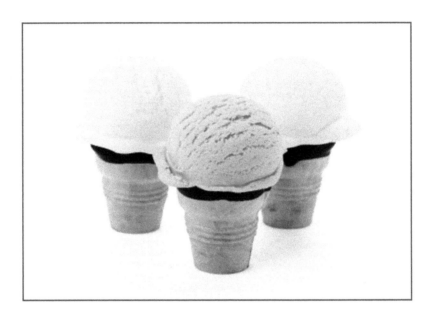

Servings:8

INGREDIENTS

- 250 G Icing sugar
- 250 ml Whole milk
- 4 Pc egg yolk
- 250 G Mascarpone
- 250 ml orange juice
- 250 ml Lemon juice
- 250 ml Clementine or mandarin juice
- 1 Tbsp Cointreau
- 0.5 TL Orange blossom water
- 750 G ripe fresh strawberries

- 1 Tbsp Fruit liqueur or dark rum
- 0.5 TL Orange blossom water
- 90 G sugar
-

PREPARATION

1. For the lemon ice cream, mix the juices, orange juice, lemon juice, clementine or tangerine juice with the liqueur and orange blossom water and strain.
2. For the strawberry ice cream, puree the strawberries with 90 g sugar, heat them in a water bath for about 10 minutes and pour them through a sieve to remove the seeds.
3. This is how you make the basis for the ice cream: Bring the milk to a boil. Beat the egg yolks and sugar to a whitish cream, slowly stir in the hot milk and stir in the water bath until it starts to become thick. Add the mascarpone spoon by spoon and stir until it is dissolved. Place the bowl in ice water to cool, stirring occasionally.
4. Mix the juice under one part of the mixture, the strawberry puree with the liqueur and orange blossom water under the others, put in the ice cream machine according to the manufacturer's instructions or freeze in covered plastic

containers. Then let thaw a little in the refrigerator for 25-40 minutes before eating.

5. If you don't have an ice cream machine, you have to freeze the ice cream in a covered plastic container.

6. This takes about 4-6 hours. Stir the mixture from the edge every hour so that it freezes evenly.

7. The structure is not that creamy, but the ice cream tastes delicious anyway.

PANNA COTTA

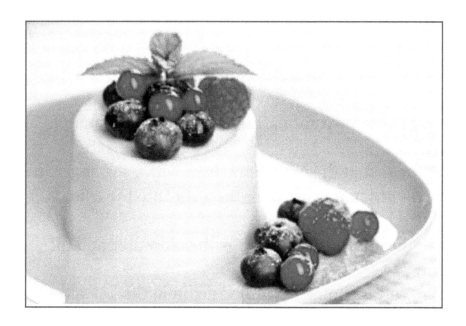

Servings:4

INGREDIENTS

- 1 Pc lemon
- 50 G sugar
- 1 Pc Vanilla pod
- 4 Bl gelatin
- 1 Tbsp Icing sugar
- 500 ml Whipped cream

PREPARATION

In a saucepan, bring 250 grams of whipped cream, vanilla pulp, sugar and a pinch of grated lemon zest to the boil.

Then take it off the stove.

Soak the gelatine in a little water, then squeeze it out and add to the saucepan while stirring constantly.

Then put the mixture in the refrigerator for about 1 hour.

Beat the rest of the whipped cream with icing sugar in a bowl until it appears stiff, then stir into the cold mixture.

Rinse the appropriate forms with cold water and fill them.

Panna cottas should be chilled again in the refrigerator for at least 2 hours.

Before serving, turn the panna cottas out onto suitable plates and refine with any sugared fruit.

CRÈME CARAMEL

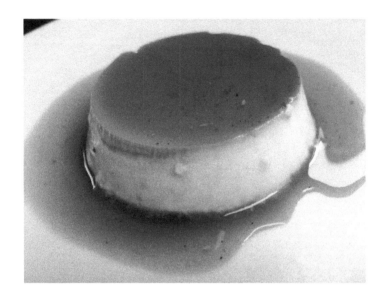

Servings:2

INGREDIENTS

- 300 G Double cream
- 2 Bl Gelatin
- 1 Tbsp Mandarin Liqueur
- 0.33 Pc from the vanilla pod (only pulp)
- 40 G sugar

PREPARATION

Soak the gelatine in cold water.

Slowly bring the crème double, pulp from the vanilla pod, tangerine liqueur and sugar to the boil.

Remove the pot from the stove and let it cool down a little.

Then add the pressed gelatine and stir well.

Pass through a fine sieve, fill into the desired molds and refrigerate.

Garnish with an orange slice and serve with orange concentrate or strawberry syrup.

GIOTTO CUTS

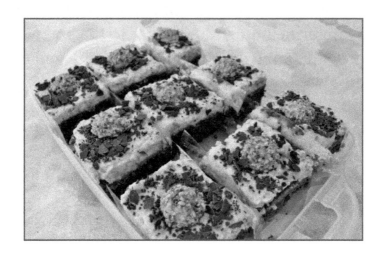

Servings:12

INGREDIENTS

- 80 G Flour
- 0.5 Pk baking powder
- 100 G butter
- 5 Pc Eggs
- 100 G Hazelnuts (grated)
- 60 G Breadcrumbs
- 100 G Icing sugar

for the cream
- 250 G butter
- 250 G Icing sugar

- 1 Pkvanilla sugar
- 4 Pc Eggs
- 250 G Hazelnuts (grated)
- 2 cups Whipped cream
- 30 Pc Giotto balls
- 1 Pk Cream stiffener
-

PREPARATION

1. Separate the eggs, stir together the yolks, butter and icing sugar until frothy.
2. Stir in the nuts, breadcrumbs and baking powder.
3. Beat egg whites into snow.
4. Carefully fold the egg whites with the flour into the yolk mixture. Spread the mixture on a baking sheet lined with baking paper and bake at 180 ° C for about 1 hour.
5. For the cream: separate eggs.
6. Mix the yolks, butter, icing sugar and vanilla sugar until frothy.
7. Beat egg whites into snow. Carefully stir the nuts with the egg white.
8. Crush approx. 30 Giotto balls with a rolling pin. Mix the whipped cream with the whipped cream and fold in the crushed Giotto balls. Add the whipped cream to the cream.

9. Spread the mixture on the cooled cake and garnish with chocolate flakes.

CREAMY PANNA COTTA

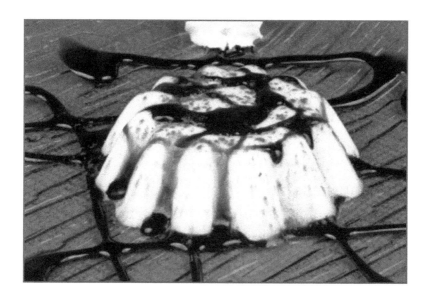

Servings:4

INGREDIENTS

- 75 G sugar
- 250 ml milk
- 250 ml Whipped cream
- 2 Pck vanilla sugar
- 3 Tr Taste of rum
- 3 Tr Vanilla flavor
- 5 Bl gelatin

PREPARATION

1. Soak gelatin in water.
2. Put the whipped cream, milk, vanilla sugar and sugar in a saucepan and bring to the boil briefly.
3. Flavor the cream with the aroma of vanilla and rum.
4. Dissolve the well-squeezed gelatin in the cream removed from the stove.
5. Pour the mixture into decorative molds and let them set completely in the refrigerator.
6. Before serving, turn out of the molds and decorate with a chocolate sauce.

PANNA COTTA WITH RASPBERRIES

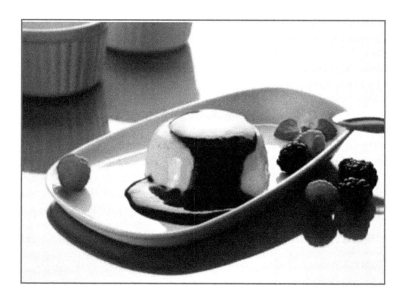

Servings:4

INGREDIENTS

- 0.06 l milk
- 40 G sugar
- 0.5 Tbsp vanilla sugar
- 0.25 l Whipped cream
- 8 Bl Gelatin
- 120 G Raspberries
- 5 G sugar
- 4 Bl mint

PREPARATION

1. Bring milk, sugar and vanilla sugar to the boil in a saucepan, then add whipped cream and bring to the boil again.
2. Soak 4 sheets of gelatine in water, squeeze out and dissolve in 2 tablespoons of water.
3. Add gelatin to the cooked mass and pour into suitable glasses that have been rinsed once.
4. Strain the raspberries, then bring to the boil with sugar and add the dissolved gelatin.
5. Then pour the raspberry sauce onto the panna cotta and place in the fridge for about 1.5 hours.
6. Refine with fresh whole raspberry pieces and mint leaves before serving.

VIENNESE ICED COFFEE

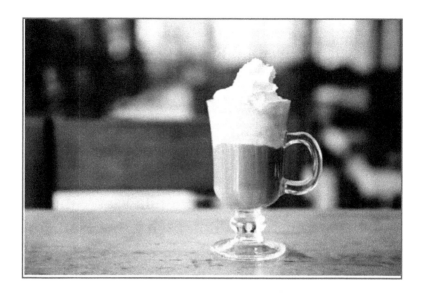

Servings:9

INGREDIENTS

- 1 l Brewed coffee (cold)
- 1 cup Whipped cream
- 1 shotAmaretto liqueur
- 60 G Sugar (brown)
- 500 G vanilla ice-cream
- 1 prize Cocoa powder
- for the decoration
- 9 Pc Amarettini

PREPARATION

1. Brew 1 liter of strong coffee in the coffee machine as usual.
2. This is now put in the cold for 2 hours.
3. The whipped cream is now whipped in a bowl with a mixer.
4. The coffee is mixed with the sugar and the amaretto and divided evenly between the glasses.
5. Now take a piece of the vanilla ice cream with a tablespoon and put it in each glass. (something dissolves very quickly)
6. Furthermore, the whipped cream comes on top, the Amarettini can be placed next to the glass as a decoration.

COCONUT PANNA COTTA

Servings:4

INGREDIENTS

- 40 cl Whipped cream
- 10 cl Semi-skimmed milk
- 100 G Grated cocoa
- 50 G sugar
- 2 Bl   Gelatin
- 1 TL   red fruit sauce

PREPARATION

1. Soak the gelatin sheets in a bowl with a little cold water.
2. Bring the whipped cream, milk, sugar and desiccated coconut to the boil in a saucepan.
3. Drain the gelatine sheets and stir the gelatine into the saucepan.
4. Remove the saucepan from the plate and mix well.
5. Rinse suitable glasses with cold water and pour the mixture into the glasses.
6. Then put in the refrigerator for about 2 hours.
7. Turn the panna cotta out of the container and garnish with a red fruit sauce before serving.

STRAWBERRY TIRAMISU FOR CHILDREN

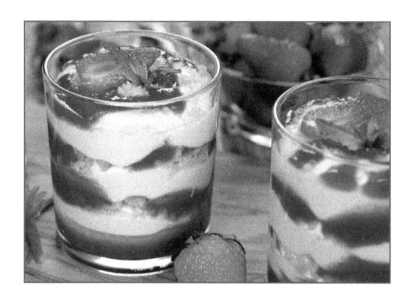

Servings:5

INGREDIENTS

- 600 G Strawberries
- 1 Pc orange
- 4 Pc   Eggs
- 70 G sugar
- 1 Pk   vanilla sugar
- 500 G Mascarpone
- 200 G Ladyfingers
- 100 G Chocolate chips

PREPARATION

1. Carefully separate the yolk and egg whites and beat the egg whites until they turn into stiff egg whites.
2. Put the egg yolks, sugar and vanilla sugar in a mixing bowl and beat everything until it is fluffy. Stir in the mascarpone.
3. Use a spatula to lift the snow into the mascarpone cream.
4. Squeeze the juice of an orange into a deep plate. Now dip one sponge cake after the other briefly into the juice and place them close together in the flat form until the bottom is completely covered.
5. Place half of the strawberries cut into pieces on the ladyfingers and spread half of the mascarpone cream on top.
6. Soak the remaining ladyfingers and place them close together on the cream. Spread the rest of the strawberries on top and cover them with the rest of the cream.
7. Put the tiramisu in the refrigerator for a few hours and sprinkle with the chocolate chips and / or strawberry puree before serving.

TIRAMISU WITH CREMEFINE WITHOUT EGG

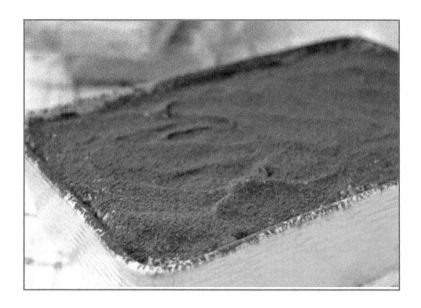

Servings:8

INGREDIENTS

- 250ml RAMA Crème fine for whipping
- 500 G Mascarpone
- 100 G Icing sugar
- 1 Pk vanilla sugar
- 1 Pc lemon
- 4 cl rum
- 0.25 lcoffee
- 60 PcBiscots (basic recipe without egg)

- 1 prize Cocoa powder for sprinkling
-

PREPARATION

1. Whip Rama Cremefine well for whipping, gradually add the sugar, vanilla sugar, a little lemon zest and a few drops of lemon juice.
2. At the end, stir in the mascarpone spoon by spoon into the cream.
3. Mix the rum and coffee, soak each of the ladyfingers briefly and line the base of a suitable dish with it.
4. The lady fingers without egg basic recipe with cream, sprinkle then again give a location ladyfingers out alternately continue until all ladyfingers consumed.
5. The final layer must consist of cream.
6. Just before serving, sprinkle thickly with cocoa.

PANNA COTTA WITH ZABAGLIONE

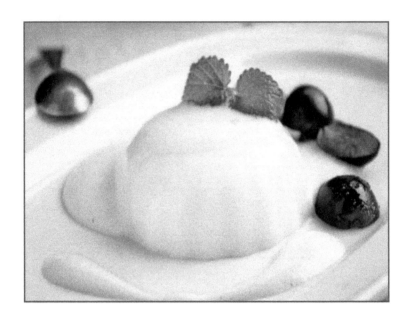

Servings:4

INGREDIENTS

- 0.5 l Whipped cream
- 4 Tbsp sugar
- 0.5 Pc Vanilla stick
- 2 Bl gelatin
- 4 Tbsp Sugar for caramel

for the zabaione cream

- 2 Pc Egg yolks
- 2 Tbsp sugar
- 100 ml Prosecco
-

PREPARATION

1. Melt the sugar for the caramel in a pan at low temperature until it is golden in color.
2. Then distribute the caramel in the molds. Warm the cream with vanilla and sugar, do not boil.
3. First put the gelatine in cold water until it is soft. Then immediately add to the cream and stir until it has completely dissolved.
4. Then fill the molds and let them cool for 6 hours.
5. Zabaione:
6. Put all the ingredients in a bowl. Now stir quickly over steam with a whisk until they become a firm foam.

BUDINO

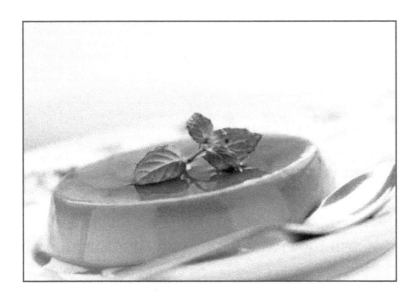

Servings:7

INGREDIENTS

- 1 Pc Vanilla pod
- 0.5 l Whipped cream
- 50 G sugar
- 4th Bl white gelatin
- fruit sauce
- 200 G sugar
- 4 Tbsp water

PREPARATION

1. Slit the vanilla pod lengthways and scrape out the pulp.
2. Bring the pod and pulp with the cream and sugar to the boil.
3. Let the gelatin soak in cold water for 10 minutes.
4. Remove the vanilla pod from the hot cream, dissolve the gently squeezed gelatine sheets in the hot cream while stirring.
5. Rinse the silicone molds with cold water, pour the cream into the molds and leave to set overnight in the refrigerator.
6. For the sauce, bring the sugar and water to the boil without stirring until the whole thing turns amber.
7. To serve, turn the panna cotta out of the molds onto a plate and pour the sauce over them.

MACEDONIA ALLO ZABAIONE

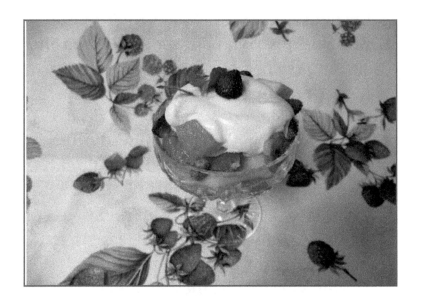

Servings:4

INGREDIENTS
- 100 G Raspberries
- 100 G Wild strawberries
- 2 Pc yellow peaches
- 6 Pc Apricots
- 1 Pc Pear (firm, ripe)
- 1 Pc Apple (sour)
- 1 Pc Lemon (juice)
- 80 G sugar
- 3 Pc egg yolk

- 125 ml dry Marsala
-

PREPARATION

1. Carefully wash the berries and pat dry.
2. Peel the peaches, cut in half, stone and cut into cubes. Wash the apricots, dry them, cut them in half, stone them and cut them into wedges. Wash and peel the pear and apple, remove the core and cut the fruit into cubes.
3. Put all the fruit in a bowl, mix with the lemon juice and about 50 g sugar.
4. Let it steep in the refrigerator for about 1 hour. Carefully turn the berries and pieces of fruit once in between.
5. In the meantime, beat the egg yolks and the remaining sugar in a heatproof bowl with a whisk or hand mixer until creamy.
6. Then place the bowl in a hot water bath, slowly pour in the Marsala and beat to a fluffy, frothy cream.
7. The wine foam must not boil.
8. It is best to place the bowl in ice-cold water and stir until the frothed wine is still lukewarm. Divide the fruit salad in portion bowls.
9. Serve the zabaione extra or pour over the fruit.

PANNA COTTA ON WILD BERRY JELLY

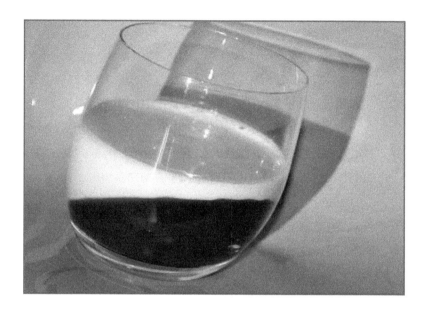

Servings:4

INGREDIENTS

- 250 ml milk
- 250 ml Whipped cream
- 1 Pc Vanilla pod
- 3 Bl gelatin
- 50 G sugar
- 200 G Wild berries
- 50 G sugar
- 20 ml Berry juice

- 2 Bl gelatin

PREPARATION

1. First, the wild berry jelly is made.
2. Soak the 2 sheets of gelatine in cold water, put the berries with 50 grams of sugar and the berry juice in a saucepan, heat slowly over a mild heat, simmer briefly and pass through a fine sieve. Heat the berry puree again and dissolve the well-squeezed gelatin in it.
3. Rinse 4 glasses with cold water and place them at an angle, for example in an egg carton, pour the fruit puree and let it set in the refrigerator.
4. For the panna cotta, slit open the vanilla pod lengthways and scrape out the pulp, soak 3 sheets of gelatine in cold water.
5. Put the cream with the milk 50 grams of sugar, the vanilla pulp and the vanilla pod in a saucepan and bring to the boil, remove from the hob, squeeze out the gelatine and dissolve in the milk cream.
6. Let the mixture cool down to room temperature and pour it into the glasses that have just been placed. Chill the panna cotta for at least 4 hours.

GINGERBREAD TIRAMISU

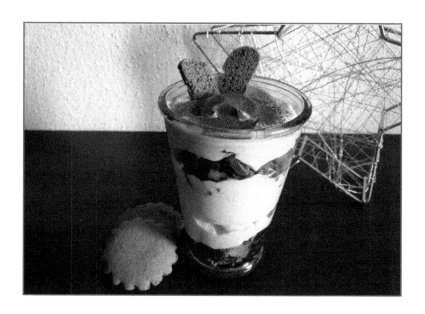

SERVINGS:6

INGREDIENTS

- 2 Pc Cloves
- 1 Tbsp Cocoa powder
- 220 G gingerbread
- 200 G Mascarpone
- 3 Tbsp milk
- 220 G Curd cheese (fine)
- 1 Pk vanilla sugar
- 200 ml red wine

- 2 Stg cinnamon
- 80 G sugar
-

PREPARATION

1. For a gingerbread tiramisu, mix the mascarpone, curd cheese, sugar, milk and vanilla sugar well in a bowl - the gingerbread is cut into strips.
2. Bring the wine, cloves and cinnamon to the boil in a saucepan and briefly dip the gingerbread in it on both sides.
3. Layer the gingerbread in any shape, spread the mascarpone cream over it and place the gingerbread on top of the cream again.
4. Repeat the process until there is no gingerbread left.
5. Finish with the curd cream.
6. Place the gingerbread tiramisu in the refrigerator for about 4-5 hours.
7. Sprinkle the cocoa powder on top before serving.

PANNA COTTA WITH ESPRESSO JELLY

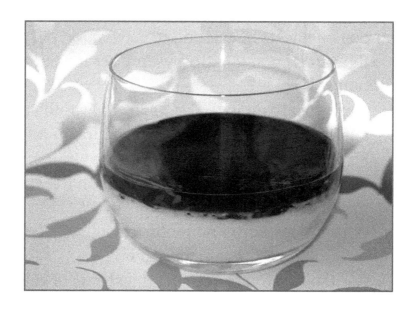

Servings:4

INGREDIENTS

- 500 G Whipped cream
- 55 G sugar
- 1 Pc Vanilla pod
- 125 ml espresso
- 2 TL sugar
- 1.5 Bl Gelatin (white)
- 4 Bl   Gelatin (white)

PREPARATION

1. Soak 4 sheets of gelatine in cold water, slit open the vanilla pod lengthways and scrape out the pulp.
2. Heat the cream with the sugar, the vanilla pod and the vanilla pulp until just before boiling, remove the vanilla pod.
3. Dissolve the well squeezed gelatin in the cream mixture.
4. Pour the mixture into molds rinsed with cold water and refrigerate for 4-6 hours.
5. For the espresso jelly, soak 1.5 sheets of gelatine in cold water, prepare 125 ml espresso and sweeten with 2 teaspoons of sugar.
6. Squeeze out the gelatine well and dissolve it in the hot espresso, let the mixture cool down as much as possible (otherwise the panna cotta would melt) divide it into the panna cotta glasses, chill for at least 1 hour and serve.

RASPBERRY TIRAMISU

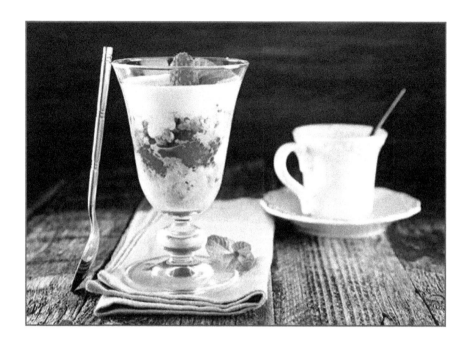

Servings:4

INGREDIENTS

- 300 G Raspberries
- 100 G Icing sugar
- 1 Pk vanilla sugar
- 0.5 Pc Lime (juice)
- 400 G Mascarpone
- 4 cl rum
- 0.25 l coffee
- 60 Pc Ladyfingers

- 500 ml Rama Cremefine for whipping
-

PREPARATION

1. First, finely puree 150 g raspberries with a hand blender.
2. Then whip Rama Cremefine well, gradually adding icing sugar, vanilla sugar, lime juice and raspberry puree
3. Then stir in the mascarpone spoon by spoon. Finally stir the remaining raspberries into the cream.
4. Now mix the rum and coffee, briefly soak the biscuits individually and layer them in the glasses.
5. Lightly press on the biscuit mixture.
6. Then top with raspberries.
7. Then add some more ladyfingers and brush with the cream.
8. Continue with the other glasses until all the ladyfingers, raspberries and cream are used up. The final layer must consist of cream.

COCONUT PANNA COTTA

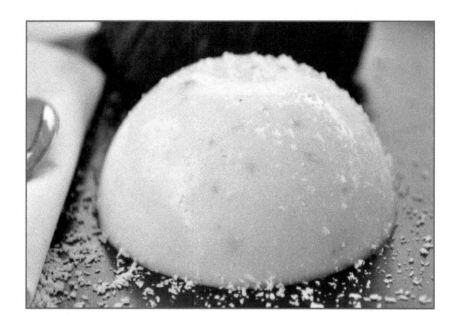

Servings:6

INGREDIENTS

- 2.5 Blgelatin
- 400 ml Coconut milk
- 250 ml Whipped cream
- 130 G Fine granulated sugar
- 0.5 Pc Limes

PREPARATION

1. Soak the gelatin sheets in cold water for 5 minutes.
2. Bring coconut milk, whipped cream and sugar to the boil in a saucepan over medium heat until the sugar dissolves, then remove from heat.
3. Squeeze out the gelatine sheets and stir them into the still warm mixture until the gelatine has dissolved.
4. Then squeeze the lime and stir in the juice.
5. Pour the finished mixture into glasses and put in the refrigerator for about 3-4 hours.

VANILLA PANNA COTTA ON A BERRY DISH

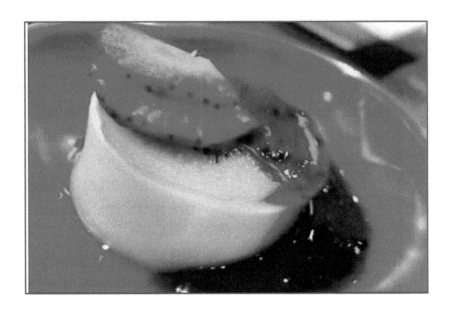

Servings:4

INGREDIENTS

- 6 Bl Gelatin (white)
- 1 Pc Vanilla pod
- 500 ml Whipped cream
- 5 Tbsp sugar
- for the berry mirror
- 220 G Strawberries
- 1 Pk vanilla sugar
- 1 Pc Kiwi (for decoration)

PREPARATION

1. For the panna cotta: score the vanilla pod and scrape out the pulp.
2. Soak the gelatine in cold water. Then bring the whipped cream, sugar, vanilla pulp including the pod to the boil in a saucepan.
3. Then remove the vanilla pod and let it cool down to lukewarm.
4. Add the squeezed gelatine and stir well.
5. Pass through a sieve, fill into the desired molds and refrigerate for at least 3 hours.
6. For the berry mirror:
7. Wash the berries, pat dry with kitchen paper if necessary, puree and season with vanilla sugar.
8. Tip the panna cotta out of the molds.
9. Arrange on plates with the pureed berry sauce and decorate with kiwi and strawberry slices.

SUMMER MELON SALAD

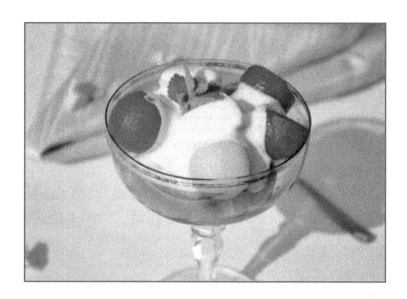

Servings:4

INGREDIENTS

- 1 Pc Watermelon
- 1 Pc Sugar melon
- 4 Tbsp Icing sugar
- 4 cl Maraschino

dressing
- 1 cups yogurt
- 3 Tbsp Lemon juice
- 2 Tbsp Icing sugar

PREPARATION

1. First peel the watermelon, remove the stones and cut out small balls from the pulp with a spherical cutter.
2. You do the same with the sugar melon.
3. Mix the melon ball well and put it in the fridge with icing sugar and maraschino for 1 hour.
4. Pour the mixed melon balls into dessert glasses and set aside.
5. For the dressing, stir the yogurt with the lemon juice and icing sugar and pour it over the melon balls.

FINE ROSEMARY ICE CREAM

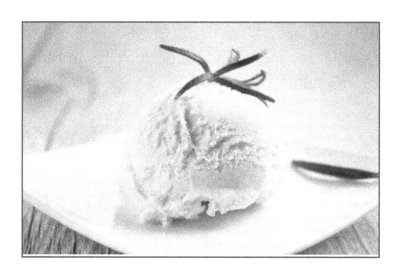

Servings:4

INGREDIENTS

- 4 Pc   Rosemary sprigs
- 300 ml Whipped cream
- 250 ml milk
- 80 G sugar
- 4 Pc Eggs
-

PREPARATION

1. Bring the rosemary with cream, milk and a pinch of the sugar to the boil and simmer for about five minutes.

2. Beat the eggs with the yolks and the remaining sugar in a bowl.
3. Pour the warm liquid over the egg mixture and carefully fold in.
4. Now just let it cool down and then freeze in the ice cream maker.

COFFEE TIRAMISU

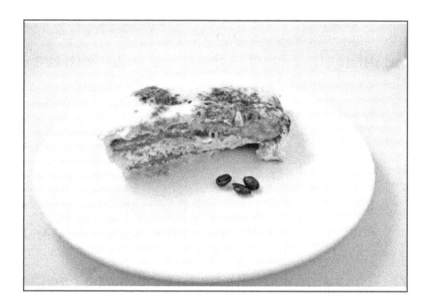

Servings:4

INGREDIENTS

- 40 Pc Ladyfingers
- 4 Tbsp Icing sugar
- 4 Pc Eggs
- 250 ml Black coffee)
- 2 Tbsp Dissolving coffee
- 500 G Mascarpone

PREPARATION

1. Beat egg whites into snow.
2. In another bowl, stir the egg yolks with the sugar until foamy, until a thick, creamy mixture is formed.
3. Alternately fold in the mascarpone and egg whites.
4. Prepare black coffee.
5. Dip one side of the ladyfingers in the coffee and cut into a rectangular shape. Then brush with the mascarpone cream.
6. Then sprinkle with half a tablespoon of coffee powder.
7. Now dip the ladyfingers in the coffee again, layer them in the mold and coat with mascarpone cream. Sprinkle again with half a tablespoon of loosing coffee.
8. Repeat the process until there is no more cream or lady fingers.
9. Finally, finish with the cream and sprinkle with a tablespoon of dissolving coffee.
   Place in the refrigerator for about 6 hours.

MOCHA CREAM

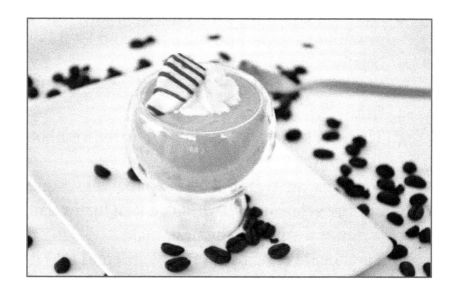

Servings:4

INGREDIENTS
- 0.5 l milk
- 4 Pc Egg yolk
- 4 Pc Egg white
- 4 Tbsp Dissolving coffee
- 40 G Granulated sugar
- 8 Bl gelatin

for decorating
- 0.125 l Whipped cream
- 20 G Mocca beans

PREPARATION

1. At the beginning, mix half of the milk with the granulated sugar and the coffee and let it boil briefly in a saucepan.
2. Mix the rest of the milk with the yolks until frothy.
3. Then soak the gelatine in cold water for about 10 minutes.
4. Now mix the two milk masses together, squeeze out the gelatine well, dissolve it in lukewarm water and stir into the milk mass.
5. Then beat the egg white until stiff and fold it into the cream that is starting to thicken.
6. Finally, pour the cream into bowls, refrigerate for 1 hour and decorate with whipped cream and mocca beans before serving.

VEGETARIAN TIRAMISU

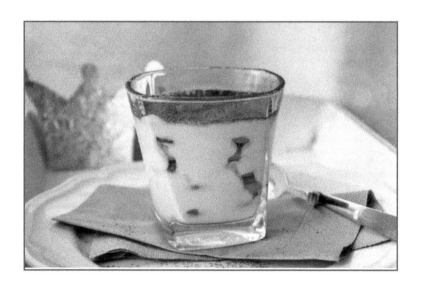

Servings:6

INGREDIENTS

- 250 mg Coffee, espresso, cold
- 1 shot Amaretto

for the dough
- 130 GFlour
- 80 G sugar
- 3 Tbsp Sunflower oil
- 130 ml water
- 2 TL baking powder
- for the cream
- 280 ml Soy cream

- 150 ml water
- 80 G sugar
- 50 G semolina
- 1 Pc BIO lemon, zest
- 1 Pk vanilla sugar
- 1 TL Cinnamon powder
- 2 Tbsp Amaretto
- 1 prize salt
- 50 G margarine
-

PREPARATION

1. For the dough, mix the sunflower oil, flour, sugar, water and baking powder well in a bowl with the mixer and spread on a baking sheet lined with baking paper (approx. 20x30 cm). Bake the dough in a preheated oven at 180 degrees (top / bottom heat) for about 20 minutes and allow to cool.
2. For the cream, mix the soy cream with the water, sugar and semolina well in a saucepan and bring to the boil briefly.
3. Now add the grated lemon zest, vanilla sugar, cinnamon, amaretto and a pinch of salt and stir everything well.
4. Chill the mixture in the refrigerator for an hour - stirring every now and then.

5. After an hour, take the mixture out of the fridge, add the room-temperature margarine and stir until a creamy mixture has formed.
6. Now mix the coffee with the amaretto and place on a plate.
7. Cut the cooled sponge cake into thin, approx. 2 cm thick strips and dip them into the coffee-amaretto mixture.
8. Place the strips on the bottom of a baking dish (20x20 cm), spread some cream over them, then another layer of biscuit strips and finally another layer of cream.
9. Put the baking dish in the refrigerator for at least 30 minutes and sprinkle with cocoa powder just before serving.

TIRAMISU MUFFINS

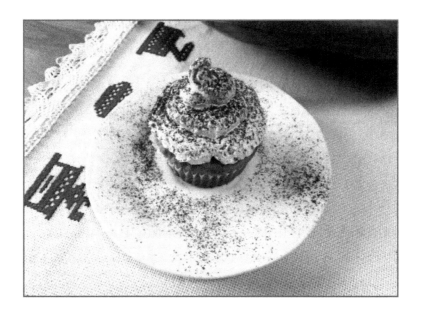

Servings:6

INGREDIENTS

- 2 Pc Eggs
- 50 G sugar
- 25 G Flour smooth)
- 25 G Maizena (cornstarch)
- 1 Tbsp Custard powder
- 0.5 TL baking powder
- 0.5 Cup espresso
- 125 G Mascarpone

- 50 G Icing sugar
- 50 ml Whipped cream
- 2 Tbsp Cocoa powder

PREPARATION

1. First of all, separate the eggs and beat the egg whites until stiff.
2. Gradually add sugar and continue beating until the mixture is glossy.
3. Then add the egg yolk and stir in.
4. Mix together the flour, cornstarch, vanilla pudding and baking powder. Pour the mixture into a sieve and sieve onto the egg mixture, then stir carefully.
5. Spread the dough evenly on the muffin tray lined with paper cases and bake for about 25 minutes at 175 ° C top / bottom heat.
6. After the muffins have been baked, they should cool completely.
7. In the meantime, brew a cup of espresso.
8. Beat the mascarpone with icing sugar until airy and stir in two tablespoons of espresso. Then whip the whipped cream until stiff and add to the mixture.
9. Drizzle the rest of the espresso over the muffins, which have previously been pierced several times with a fork. Then the mascarpone cream is spread over the muffins with a piping bag.

HOMEMADE STRAWBERRY ICE CREAM

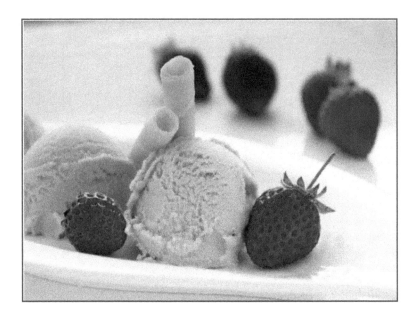

Servings:6

INGREDIENTS

- 0.5 l milk
- 0.5 l Whipped cream
- 150 G sugar
- 200 G Strawberries
- 10 Pc Egg yolk

PREPARATION

1. Bring the yolks to the boil with cold milk, sugar and whipped cream.
2. Puree the strawberries and add to the hot milk-cream mixture.
3. Now add the yolk mixture to the mass, then heat with constant stirring (the mass will be slightly creamy), but not above 80 ° C; otherwise the mixture will become crumbly.
4. Now place the bowl in a prepared ice water bath to quickly cool the mass.
5. Stir in an ice cream maker for 35 minutes.
6. If you don't have an ice cream machine: Pour the mixture into a chrome steel bowl, freeze it at -18 degrees and stir with a whisk every 10 minutes.
7. The strawberry ice cream is ready after 1 1/2 to 2 hours.

TUSCAN CANTUCCI

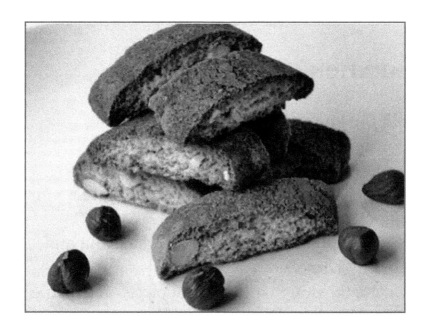

Servings: 40

INGREDIENTS

- 130 G Flour
- 0.5 TL baking powder
- 90 G sugar
- 1 Pk vanilla sugar
- 1 prize salt
- 20 G grated marzipan paste
- 15 G Butter (soft)
- 1 Pc egg

- 50 G Almond kernels
- 40 G Hazelnut kernels
- 0.5 TL gingerbread spice
-

PREPARATION

1. Sift the flour into a bowl with the baking powder, sugar, vanilla sugar, gingerbread spices, 1 pinch of salt, the egg and the soft butter with a dough hook and knead into a smooth dough.
2. Knead in the marzipan mixture, hazelnut and almond kernels.
3. Divide the dough into 2 equal pieces and shape into rolls, wrap them in cling film and refrigerate for 2 hours.
4. Preheat the oven to 180 ° C and line a baking sheet with parchment paper.
5. Pre-bake the rolls of dough with enough space on the middle rack for about 15 minutes.
6. Let the rolls cool down and cut into approx. 1 cm thick slices, place the cantucci on the baking sheet and bake again at 180 ° C for 10-12 minutes until golden brown.
7. Let the cantucci cool on a wire rack.

STEVIA STRAWBERRY ICE CREAM

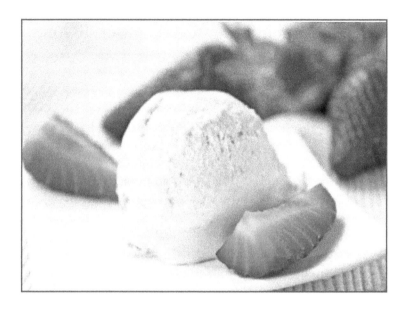

Servings:4

INGREDIENTS

- 250 G Strawberries
- 125 G Whipped cream
- 3 Tbsp milk
- 2 Tbsp Lemon juice
- 0.25 TL Stevioside powder (white)

for the garnish
- 8 Pc Strawberries

PREPARATION

1. First mix milk and stevia in a saucepan and only heat until the stevia powder dissolves. then let it cool down. In the meantime, puree the strawberries.
2. Now stir the milk with lemon juice into the strawberry puree and pass everything through a fine sieve to remove the stones.
3. Then whip the whipped cream until stiff and stir into the strawberry-milk mixture, season to taste again and add stevia powder if necessary (note: the mixture tastes less sweet when frozen).
4. Finally, pour the mixture into an ice cream maker and let it freeze for about 20 minutes. Serve garnished with strawberries.

MANGOTIRAMISU

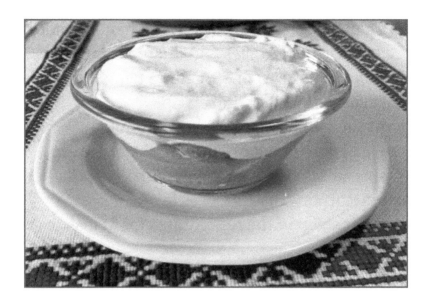

Servings:8

INGREDIENTS

- 1 Pc   mango
- 2 Pc   Oranges
- 250 G Mascarpone
- 25 Pc Ladyfingers
- 180 ml yogurt
- 180 ml Whipped cream
- 75 G sugar
- 1 Pk vanilla sugar

PREPARATION

1. Peel the mango and cut into cubes.
2. Then process into puree with a hand blender. Squeeze the oranges and dip the biscuits.
3. Mix the mascarpone, yogurt, sugar and vanilla sugar with a hand mixer.
4. At the end, whip the cream and fold in.
5. Place the dipped biscuits in a baking dish, spread the puree on top and finally spread the mascarpone mixture over it.
6. Let it steep in the refrigerator for at least 2 hours.

PANNA COTTA WITH NUTS

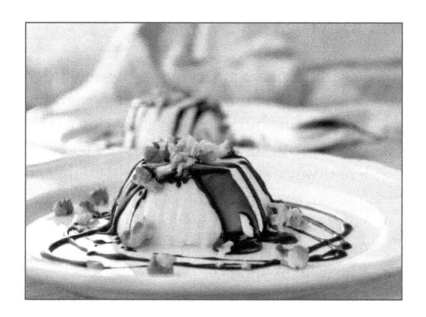

Servings:4

INGREDIENTS

- 4 Tbsp Peanut butter
- 400 ml Almond milk
- 50 mlAgave syrup
- 0.5 TL Agar Agar
- 1 Pc Vanilla pod
- for the chocolate sauce
- 100 G Chocolate, dark, vegan
- 100 ml water
- 3 TL Cocoa powder
- 1 TL sugar

- 2 Tbsp Nuts, chopped
-

PREPARATION

1. For the panna cotta, first put the almond milk in a saucepan, mix well with the peanut butter, agave syrup and agar agar and bring to the boil.
2. In the meantime, score the vanilla pod lengthways, scrape out the vanilla pulp and place in the saucepan.
3. Let the mixture simmer gently for a good 50 minutes - stirring again and again.
4. Rinse small molds or bowls with cold water and pour the hot panna cotta mixture into the molds.
5. Cover and place in the refrigerator for at least 3 hours.
6. For the chocolate sauce, finely chop the chocolate.
7. Bring the water to a boil in a saucepan, stir in the cocoa powder, sugar and chocolate pieces and process into a smooth mass.
8. Turn the solidified panna cotta out of the shells, pour the chocolate sauce over it lightly and decorate with finely chopped nuts.

ZABAIONE

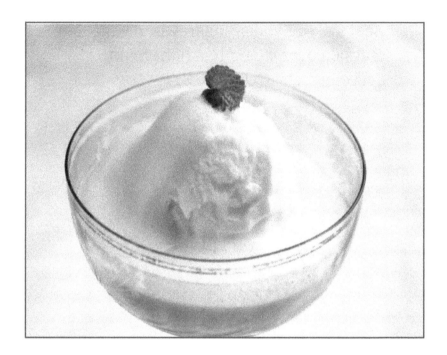

Servings:4

INGREDIENTS

- 2 Pc egg yolk
- 80 G sugar
- 100 ml White wine
- 100 ml Marsala
- 4 Bullet ice

PREPARATION

1. Beat the egg yolks, sugar, white wine and marsala over steam to a light foam.
2. Serve in a glass with ice.

PANETTONE

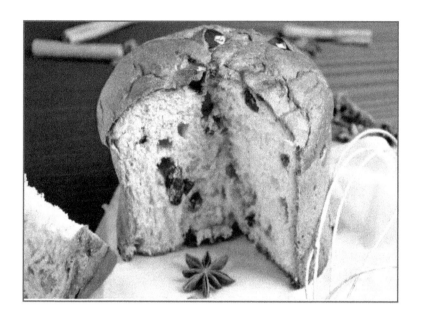

Servings:12

INGREDIENTS

- 450 G Flour
- 120 Gsugar
- 125 ml milk
- 1 Wf yeast
- 2 Tbsp Butter, for greasing
- 1 prize salt
- 1 Pk Orange peel
- 6 Pc Eggs
- 200 G Raisins

- 200 G butter
- 80 G Cherries, candied
-

PREPARATION

1. Work the flour, yeast, milk and salt into a firm dough.
2. Cover and let rise for 15 minutes.
3. Add eggs, butter and salt and knead again well.
4. Mix the orange peel, candied cherries and raisins and work into the dough.
5. Grease the cake tin with butter and pour in the batter.
6. Cover and let rise for 20 minutes.
7. Bake in the preheated oven at 220 degrees on the lowest rack for 60 minutes.
8. Halfway through the baking time, brush the cake with melted butter.

TIRAMISU - AMARETTO AND ALMOND SLIVERS

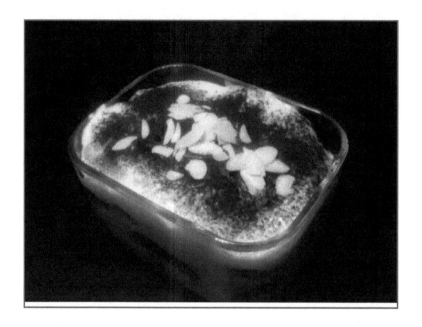

Servings:4

INGREDIENTS

- 1 Cup Black coffee)
- 2 Tbsp sugar
- 40 ml Amaretto / almond liqueur
- 4 Pc Eggs
- 100 G sugar
- 1 prize salt
- 500 G Mascarpone
- 1 Pk Ladyfingers

- 150 G almonds
-

PREPARATION

1. Brew a cup of coffee with 2 tablespoons of sugar.
2. Mix 1-2 stamperl Amaretto (omit for children of course) and let cool.
3. Separate 4 eggs and beat the egg white with a pinch of salt.
4. Mix the yolks with 100 g sugar. Stir in 1 pack of mascarpone (500g).
5. Fold in snow.
6. Unpack 1 whole pack (i.e. there are 2 packs in one box, thus both packs).
7. Pour the cold coffee mixture into a soup plate. Prepare one large bowl or many small bowls.
8. Dip only 2 sponge fingers at a time and put one layer on each bowl.
9. Mascarpone cream on top and again a layer of dipped ladyfingers, a layer of almond slivers and and finish with a layer of mascarpone cream.
   Cover with cling film and refrigerate for at least 6 hours. Then sprinkle with cocoa and enjoy in a spoonful.

OLIVE OIL CAKE

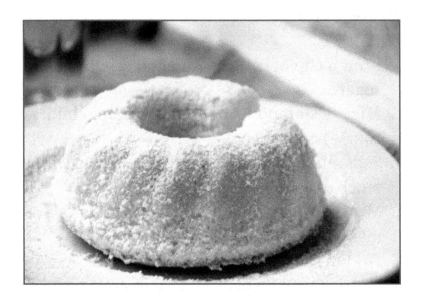

Servings:1

INGREDIENTS

- 120 GFlour
- 110 G sugar
- 40 G egg yolk
- 25 G Lemon juice
- 0.5 Pc Organic lemon (zest of it)
- 4 G Vanilla pulp
- 160 G olive oil
- 100 G Egg white (chilled)
- 1 prize salt

- 60 G sugar
-

PREPARATION

1. First sift the flour and preheat the oven to 165 ° C.
2. Then beat the sugar, egg yolk, lemon juice, lemon zest and the vanilla pulp in a mixing bowl until creamy.
3. Then carefully stir in the sifted flour and then very slowly pour in the olive oil.
4. Now, in a metal bowl, whip half the egg white, then add salt and sugar and continue to beat until it is still creamy.
5. Now fold this under 3 times under the egg yolk and flour mixture.
6. Now grease a springform pan (20 cm), sprinkle with breadcrumbs and finally pour in the mixture.
7. Now into the oven.
8. The length of the cake varies depending on the oven.
9. It is best to test with the needle sample whether the cake is ready.

PANNA COTTA WITH FIGS

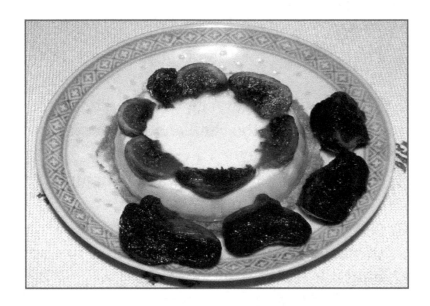

Servings:4

INGREDIENTS

- 0.5 l Whipped cream
- 150 G sugar
- 0.5 Stg Vanilla pod
- 4 Bl   gelatin
- 12 Pc Figs
- 300 ml port wine
- 1 Pc Cinnamon stick
- 1 Pc Lemon peel
- 4 Pc Cloves

- 3 Pc Eggs
- 60 G sugar
- 50 G Flour smooth)
- 20 G butter

PREPARATION

1. Preheat the oven to 180 ° C top / bottom heat. Beat eggs and sugar in a bowl until frothy.
2. Mix in the melted butter and flour.
3. Line a baking sheet with parchment paper and spread the biscuit mixture 1 cm thick. Bake the sponge cake in the oven for about 15 minutes. Then loosen the biscuit mixture and divide it into smaller pieces.
4. In a bowl, mix the whipped cream, the pulp of the vanilla pod and sugar and cook for 15 minutes.
5. Let simmer over medium heat. Soak the gelatine in cold water.
6. In the meantime, let the whipped cream cool down a bit, then stir it into the gelatine. Rinse suitable cups with cold water and fill with the mixture.
7. Then put in the refrigerator for about 30 minutes.
8. Remove the fig stalks. Heat the sugar and figs in a saucepan, stirring constantly. Pour the

whole with port wine and add the cloves and
cinnamon sticks.

9. Cover the figs with water and simmer for about
15 minutes over medium heat.
Then strain the figs and let them cool.
Divide the biscuit pieces on serving plates and
drizzle with the fig juice.
Tip the panna cotta from the refrigerator into
the center of the plate and place the figs on top.

VANILLA TIRAMISU

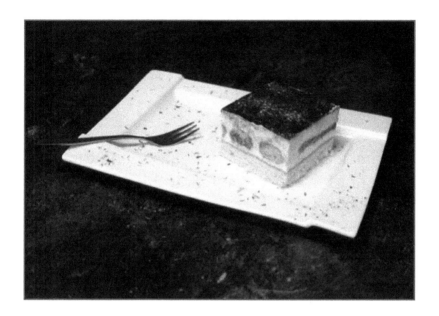

Servings:20

INGREDIENTS

- 6 Pc Eggs
- 180 G sugar
- 1 Pk vanilla sugar
- 180 G Flour

For the cream
- 1 Pk Vanilla qimiq
- 2 cups Vanilla yogurt
- 500 ml Whipped cream
- 100 G Icing sugar

- 3 Bl gelatin

For dipping
- 1 Pk Ladyfingers
- 4 clAmaretto
- 1 CupCoffee, strong

PREPARATION

1. For the dough, beat the eggs, sugar and vanilla sugar until frothy. Stir the flour into the egg mixture.
2. Spread the dough on a baking sheet lined with baking paper and bake in the preheated oven for about 18 minutes. Cover the sponge cake base with the baking frame.
3. For the cream, stir the Qimiq in a bowl until smooth. Stir in powdered sugar and vanilla yogurt. Soak the gelatine in cold water, squeeze it out, dissolve it in 1 tablespoon of hot water and stir it into the Qimiq mixture.
4. Beat the whipped cream until stiff and fold into the mixture.
5. Spread half of the cream on the sponge cake base.
6. Mix the amaretto and coffee.
7. Briefly infuse the ladyfingers and place on the cream.
8. Spread the rest of the cream on top, sprinkle with cocoa powder and refrigerate overnight.

RICOTTA CASSEROLE WITH BERRIES

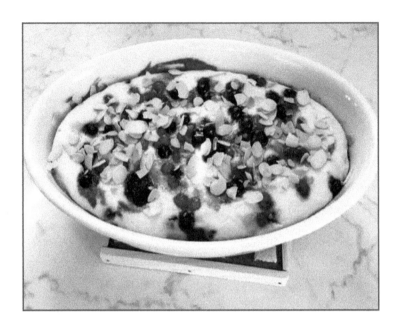

Servings: 2

INGREDIENTS

- 2 Pc Eggs, small
- 375 Gricotta
- 0.25 kg Berries, mixed
- 90 G Icing sugar
- 0.0625 kg butter
- 2 Tbsp semolina
- 0.5 Pc orange
- 0.5 Pc Lemon, zest

- 1 Tbsp almonds

PREPARATION

1. First grease 1 ovenproof dish (20 x 20), let the butter warm up at room temperature, preheat the oven at 150 ° C with a fan oven.
2. Now cut the orange into fillets, separate the eggs and beat the clear with a pinch of salt until stiff, gradually stirring in about ⅓ of the sugar. Mix the butter with the yolk, lemon zest and remaining sugar until frothy.
3. Then fold in the ricotta, semolina and finally the snow and pour half of the mixture into the molds, then spread the orange fillets and half of the berries over them.
4. Pour in the rest of the ricotta mixture and cover with some of the berries.
5. Bake everything for a maximum of 45 minutes.
6. Before the end of the cooking time, roast the almond slivers in a non-fat frying pan.
7. Sprinkle the finished casserole with slivers and the remaining berries and serve.

HALLOWEEN PANNA COTTA

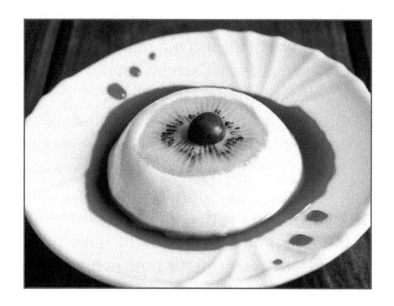

Servings:4

INGREDIENTS

- 500 G Whipped cream
- 1 Pc Vanilla pod
- 2 Bl gelatin
- 50 G sugar
- 4 Tbsp Cherry jelly
- 1 Pc kiwi
- 4 Pc Raisins

PREPARATION

1. First you prepare the panna cotta, as it has to cool for a while.
2. This can be done the day before, so that the Halloween panna cotta pulls overnight. To do this, you put the whipped cream in a tall saucepan, boil the whole thing up once and let it simmer gently.
3. The vanilla pod is halved and the vanilla pulp is scraped out with a knife, which is added to the warmed whipped cream along with the vanilla pod and sugar.
4. In the meantime, soak the gelatin in water, which should steep for 10 minutes.
5. Then take the pan off the stove, take out the vanilla pod and add the squeezed gelatine until it dissolves.
6. Then you fill the panna cotta in hot rinsed glasses and let them cool for at least 4 hours.
7. The cherry jelly is briefly heated in a saucepan so that it becomes liquid.
8. Then you give it to cool down on a plate, where you are welcome to splash something.
9. This creates the impression that it is real blood - of course you can also use simple strawberry jam for it.
   In the meantime you check whether the panna cotta has set. It should have a consistency like

pudding and give slightly. The firm panna cotta is poured onto the prepared plate and a kiwi slice is placed on top.

CONCLUSIONS

A vegetarian diet focuses on eating vegetables. This includes dried fruits, vegetables, peas and beans, grains, seeds, and nuts. There is no single type of vegetarian diet.

Vegetarian diets continue to grow in popularity. The reasons for following a vegetarian diet are varied and include health benefits, such as reduced risk of heart disease, diabetes, and some types of cancer. However, some vegetarians consume too many processed foods, which can be high in calories, sugar, fat, and sodium, and may not consume enough fruits, vegetables, whole grains, and foods rich in calcium, missing out on the nutrients they provide.

However, with a little planning, a vegetarian diet can meet the needs of people of all ages, including children, adolescents, and pregnant or lactating women. The key is to be aware of your own nutritional needs so that you can plan a diet that meets them.

Vegan diets exclude beef, chicken, and fish, eggs, and dairy products, as well as foods that contain these products. Some people follow a semi-vegetarian diet (also called a flexitarian diet) which is primarily a plant-based diet but includes meat, dairy, eggs, chicken, and fish occasionally or in small amounts. How to plan a healthy vegetarian diet

To get the most out of a vegetarian diet, choose a good variety of healthy plant foods, such as whole fruits and vegetables, legumes, nuts, and whole grains. At the same time, cut down on less healthy options like sugar-sweetened beverages, fruit juices, and refined grains. If you need help, a registered dietitian can help you create a vegetarian plan that is right for you.

To get started

One way to transition to a vegetarian diet is to progressively reduce the meat in your diet while increasing your consumption of fruits and vegetables. Here are a couple of tips to help you get started:

Gradual transition. Increase the number of meatless meals you already enjoy each week, like spaghetti with tomato sauce or stir-fry vegetables. Find ways to include vegetables, such as spinach, kale, chard, and collards, in your daily meals.

Replacements. Take your favorite recipes and try them without meat. For example, make vegetarian chili by omitting the ground beef and adding an extra can of black beans. Or make fajitas using extra firm tofu instead of chicken. You will be surprised to find that many chainrings only require simple replacements.

Diversity. Buy or borrow vegetarian cookbooks. Visit ethnic restaurants to try new vegetarian recipes. The more variety your vegetarian diet has, the more likely you are to meet all of your nutritional needs.

The vegetarian diet, if it is prepared by choosing the foods appropriately and taking into account the guidelines and indications of the doctor or nutritionist, is able to provide the body with the nutrients it needs and to ensure the maintenance of a good state of health.